CW00571301

The Ultimate Keto Chaffle Cookbook Recipes for Beginners

The Latest Recipes to Enjoy every Keto Diet and Lose Weight Fast

Veronica Lang

contained within this document, including, but not limited to, — errors, omissions, or inaccuracies.

Table of contents

Japanese Breakfast Chaffle

Servings: 2

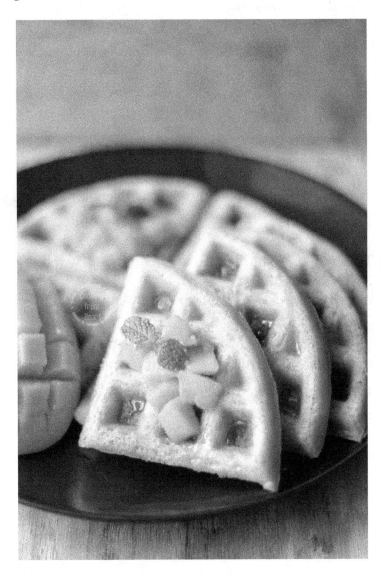

Prep time: 5 min. Cook time: 10 min.

Ingredients:

1 egg

½ cup shredded mozzarella cheese

1 Tbsp kewpie mayo

1 stalk of green onion, chopped

1 slice bacon, chopped

Directions:

Turn on waffle maker to heat and oil it with cooking spray. Beat egg in a small bowl.

Add 1 Tbsp mayo, bacon, and ½ green onion. Mix well.

Place ⅛ cup of cheese on waffle maker, then spread half of the egg mixture over it and top with ⅛ cup cheese.

Close and cook for 3-4 minutes. Repeat for remaining batter. Transfer to a plate and sprinkle with remaining green onion. Nutrition Value per Servings:

Carbs - 1 G Fat - 16 G Protein - 8 G Calories – 183

Scallion Cream Cheese Chaffle

Servings: 2

Prep time: 15 min. + 1 h. Cook time: 20 min.

Ingredients:

1 large egg

½ cup of shredded mozzarella

2 Tbsp cream cheese

1 Tbsp everything bagel seasoning

 1-2 sliced scallions

Directions:

Turn on waffle maker to heat and oil it with cooking spray. Beat egg in a small bowl.

Add in ½ cup mozzarella.

Pour half of the mixture into the waffle maker and cook for 3-4 minutes. Remove chaffle and repeat with remaining mixture.

Let them cool, then cover each chaffle with cream cheese, sprinkle with seasoning and scallions.

Nutrition Value per Servings:

Carbs - 8 G Fat - 11 G Protein - 5 G Calories – 168

Grilled Cheese Chaffle

Servings: 1

Prep time: 10 min. Cook time: 10 min.

Ingredients:

1   large egg

½ cup mozzarella cheese

2   slices yellow American cheese

2-3 slices cooked bacon, cut in half

1 tsp butter

½ tsp baking powder

Directions:

Turn on waffle maker to heat and oil it with cooking spray.

Beat egg in a bowl.

Add mozzarella, and baking powder.

Pour half of the mix into the waffle maker and cook for 4 minutes. Remove and repeat to make the second chaffle.

Layer bacon and cheese slices in between two chaffles.

Melt butter in a skillet and add chaffle sandwich to the pan. Fry on each side for 2-3 minutes covered, until cheese has melted.

Slice in half on a plate and serve. Nutrition Value per Servings:

Carbs - 4 G Fat - 18 G Protein - 7 G Calories - 233

Lemony Fresh Herbs Chaffles

Servings: 6

Cooking Time: 24 Minutes

Ingredients:

½ cup ground flaxseed

2 organic eggs

½ cup goat cheddar cheese, grated

2-4 tablespoons plain Greek yogurt

1 tablespoon avocado oil

½ teaspoon baking soda

1   teaspoon fresh lemon juice

2   tablespoons fresh chives, minced

1 tablespoon fresh basil, minced

½ tablespoon fresh mint, minced

¼ tablespoon fresh thyme, minced

¼ tablespoon fresh oregano, minced

Salt and freshly ground black pepper, to taste

Directions:

1. Preheat a waffle iron and then grease it.

2. In a medium bowl, place all ingredients and with a fork, mix until well combined.

3. Divide the mixture into 6 portions.

4. Place 1 portion of the mixture into preheated waffle iron and cook for about minutes or until golden brown.

5. Repeat with the remaining mixture.

6. Serve warm.

Nutrition value per Servings:

Calories: 11 Fat: 7.9g Carbohydrates: 3.7g Sugar: 0.7gProtein: 6.4g

Basil Chaffles

Servings: 3

Cooking Time: 16 Minutes

Ingredients:

2 organic eggs, beaten

½ cup Mozzarella cheese, shredded

1 tablespoon Parmesan cheese, grated

1 teaspoon dried basil, crushed

Pinch of salt

Directions:

1.   Preheat a mini waffle iron and then grease it.

2.   In a medium bowl, place all ingredients and mix until well combined.

3.   Place 1/of the mixture into preheated waffle iron and cook for about 3-4 minutes or until golden brown.

4.   Repeat with the remaining mixture.

5.   Serve warm.

Nutrition value per Servings:

Calories: 99 Fat: 4.2g Carbohydrates: 0.4g Sugar: 0.2g Protein: 5.7g

Scallion Cream Cheese Chaffle

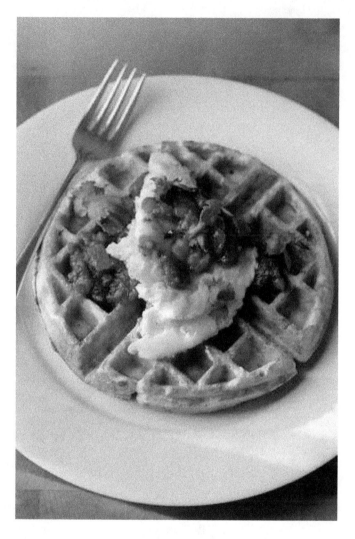

Servings: 2

Cooking Time: 20 Minutes

Ingredients:

1 large egg

½ cup of shredded mozzarella 2 Tbsp cream cheese

1 Tbsp everything bagel seasoning 1-2 sliced scallions

Directions:

1.   Turn on waffle maker to heat and oil it with cooking spray.

2.   Beat egg in a small bowl.

3.   Add in ½ cup mozzarella.

4.   Pour half of the mixture into the waffle maker and cook for 3-minutes.

5.   Remove chaffle and repeat with remaining mixture.

6.   Let them cool, then cover each chaffle with cream cheese, sprinkle with seasoning and scallions.

Nutrition value:

Carbs: 8 g ;Fat: 11 g ;Protein: 5 g ;Calories: 168

Chicken Taco Chaffles

Servings: 2

Cooking Time: 8 Minutes

Ingredients:

1/3 cup cooked grass-fed chicken, chopped 1 organic egg

1/3 cup Monterrey Jack cheese, shredded ¼ teaspoon taco seasoning

Directions:

1.   Preheat a mini waffle iron and then grease it.

2.   In a bowl, place all the ingredients and mix until well combined.

3.   Place half of the mixture into preheated waffle iron and cook for about 4 minutes or until golden brown.

4.   Repeat with the remaining mixture.

5.   Serve warm.

Nutrition value per Servings:

Calories: 141 Fat: 8.9g Carbohydrates:1.1g Sugar: 0.2g Protein: 13.5g

Crab Chaffles

Servings: 6

Cooking Time: 25 Minutes

Ingredients:

1   lb crab meat

1/3 cup Panko breadcrumbs 1 egg

2   tbsp fat greek yogurt 1 tsp Dijon mustard

2 tbsp parsley and chives, fresh 1 tsp Italian seasoning

1   lemon, juiced

Directions:

Salt, pepper to taste Add the meat. Mix well.

Form the mixture into round patties. Cook 1 patty for 3 minutes.

Remove it and repeat the process with the remaining crab chaffle mixture. Once ready, remove and enjoy warm.

Nutrition value:

Calories 99 ; Fats: 8 g ; Carbs: 4 g ; Protein: 16 g

Bacon & Egg Chaffles

Servings: 2

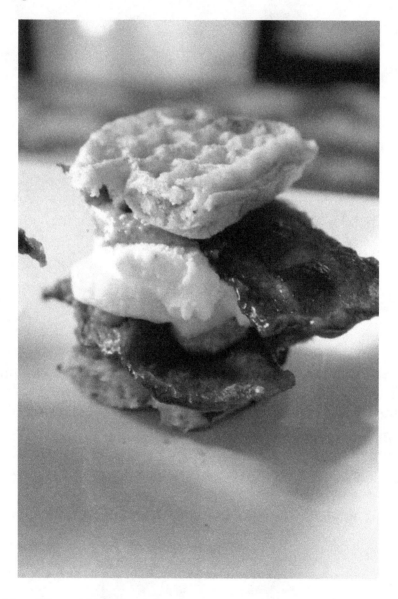

Cooking Time: 10 Minutes

Ingredients:

2 eggs

4 tsp collagen peptides, grass-fed 2 tbsp pork panko

3 slices crispy bacon

Directions:

1. Warm up your mini waffle maker.

2. Combine the eggs, pork panko, and collagen peptides. Mix well. Divide the batter in two small bowls.

3. Once done, evenly distribute ½ of the crispy chopped bacon on the waffle maker.

4. Pour one bowl of the batter over the bacon. Cook for 5 minutes and immediately repeat this step for the second chaffle.

5. Plate your cooked chaffles and sprinkle with extra Panko for an added crunch.

6. Enjoy! Nutrition value:

Calories : 266 ; Fats: 1g ; Carbs: 11.2 g ; Protein: 27 g

Chicken & Bacon Chaffles

Servings: 2

Cooking Time: 8 Minutes

Ingredients:

1   organic egg, beaten

1/3 cup grass-fed cooked chicken, chopped 1 cooked bacon slice, crumbled

1/3 cup Pepper Jack cheese, shredded 1 teaspoon powdered ranch dressing Directions:

1.   Preheat a mini waffle iron and then grease it.

2.   In a medium bowl, place all ingredients and with a fork, mix until well combined.

3.   Place half of the mixture into preheated waffle iron and cook for about 4 minutes or until golden brown.

4.   Repeat with the remaining mixture.

5.   Serve warm.

Nutrition value per Servings:

Calories: 145 Fat: 9.4g Carbohydrates: 1g Sugar: 0.2g Protein: 14.3g

Belgium Chaffles

Servings: 1

Cooking Time: 6 Minutes

Ingredients:

2   eggs

1 cup Reduced-fat Cheddar cheese, shredded

Directions:

1.   Turn on waffle maker to heat and oil it with cooking spray.

2.   Whisk eggs in a bowl, add cheese. Stir until well-combined.

3.   Pour mixture into waffle maker and cook for 6 minutes until done.

4.   Let it cool a little to crisp before serving. Nutrition value:

Carbs: 2 g ;Fat: 33 g ;Protein: 44 g ;Calories: 460

Chaffle Katsu Sandwich

Servings: 4

Cooking Time: 00 Minutes

Ingredients:

For the chicken:

¼ lb boneless and skinless chicken thigh

⅛ tsp salt

⅛ tsp black pepper

½ cup almond flour 1 egg

3 oz unflavored pork rinds

2 cup vegetable oil for deep frying For the brine:

2 cup of water 1 Tbsp salt For the sauce:

2 Tbsp sugar-free ketchup

1½ Tbsp Worcestershire Sauce 1 Tbsp oyster sauce

1   tsp swerve/monkfruit For the chaffle:

2   egg

1 cup shredded mozzarella cheese

Directions:

1. Add brine ingredients in a large mixing bowl.

2. Add chicken and brine for 1 hour.

3. Pat chicken dry with a paper towel. Sprinkle with salt and pepper. Set aside.

4. Mix ketchup, oyster sauce, Worcestershire sauce, and swerve in a small mixing bowl.

5. Pulse pork rinds in a food processor, making fine crumbs.

6. Fill one bowl with flour, a second bowl with beaten eggs, and a third with crushed pork rinds.

7. Dip and coat each thigh in: flour, eggs, crushed pork rinds. Transfer on holding a plate.

8. Add oil to cover ½ inch of frying pan. Heat to 375°F.

9. Once oil is hot, reduce heat to medium and add chicken. Cooking time

depends on the chicken thickness.

10. Transfer to a drying rack.

11. Turn on waffle maker to heat and oil it with cooking spray.

12. Beat egg in a small bowl.

13. Place ⅛ cup of cheese on waffle maker, then add¼ of the egg mixture and top with ⅛ cup of cheese.

14. Cook for 3-4 minutes.

15. Repeat for remaining batter.

16. Top chaffles with chicken katsu, 1 Tbsp sauce, and another piece of chaffle.

Nutrition value:

Carbs: 12 g ;Fat: 1 g ;Protein: 2 g ;Calories: 57

Pork Rind Chaffles

Servings: 2

Cooking Time: 10 Minutes

Ingredients:

1 organic egg, beaten

½ cup ground pork rinds

1/3 cup Mozzarella cheese, shredded Pinch of salt

Directions:

1.   Preheat a mini waffle iron and then grease it.

2.   In a bowl, place all the ingredients and beat until well combined.

3.   Place half of the mixture into preheated waffle iron and cook for about 5 minutes or until golden brown.

4.   Repeat with the remaining mixture.

5.   Serve warm.

Nutrition value per Servings:

Calories: 91 Fat: 5.9g Carbohydrates: 0.3g Sugar: 0.2g Protein: 9.2g

Chicken & Ham Chaffles

Servings: 4

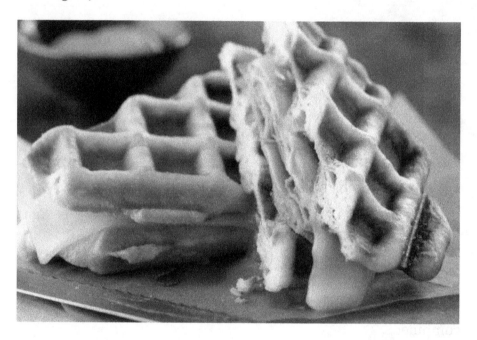

Cooking Time: 16 Minutes

Ingredients:

¼ cup grass-fed cooked chicken, chopped 1 ounce sugar-free ham, chopped

1   organic egg, beaten

¼ cup Swiss cheese, shredded

¼ cup Mozzarella cheese, shredded

Directions:

1.   Preheat a mini waffle iron and then grease it.

2.   In a medium bowl, place all ingredients and mix until well combined.

3.   Place ¼ of the mixture into preheated waffle iron and cook for about 4 minutes or until golden brown.

4.   Repeat with the remaining mixture.

5.   Serve warm.

Nutrition value per Servings:

Calories: 71 Fat: 4.2g Carbohydrates: 0.8g Sugar: 0.2g Protein: 7.4g

Eggs Benedict Chaffle

Servings: 2

Cooking Time: 10 Minutes

Ingredients:

For the chaffle:

2   egg whites

2 Tbsp almond flour 1 Tbsp sour cream

½ cup mozzarella cheese For the hollandaise:

½ cup salted butter 4 egg yolks

2 Tbsp lemon juice For the poached eggs:

2 eggs

1 Tbsp white vinegar 3 oz deli ham Directions:

1.   Whip egg white until frothy, then mix in remaining ingredients.

2.   Turn on waffle maker to heat and oil it with cooking spray.

3.   Cook for 7 minutes until golden brown.

4.   Remove chaffle and repeat with remaining batter.

5. Fill half the pot with water and bring to a boil.

6. Place heat-safe bowl on top of pot, ensuring bottom doesn't touch the boiling water.

7. Heat butter to boiling in a microwave.

8. Add yolks to double boiler bowl and bring to boil.

9. Add hot butter to the bowl and whisk briskly. Cook until the egg yolk mixture has thickened.

10. Remove bowl from pot and add in lemon juice. Set aside.

11. Add more water to pot if needed to make the poached eggs (water should completely cover the eggs). Bring to a simmer. Add white vinegar to water.

12. Crack eggs into simmering water and cook for 1 minute 30 seconds. Remove using slotted spoon.

13. Warm chaffles in toaster for 2-3 minutes. Top with ham, poached eggs, and hollandaise sauce.

Nutrition value:

Carbs: 4 g ;Fat: 26 g ;Protein: 26 g ;Calories: 365

Chicken & Veggies Chaffles

Servings: 3

Cooking Time: 15 Minutes

Ingredients:

1/3 cup cooked grass-fed chicken, chopped 1/3 cup cooked spinach, chopped

1/3 cup marinated artichokes, chopped 1 organic egg, beaten

1/3 cup Mozzarella cheese, shredded 1 ounce cream cheese, softened

¼ teaspoon garlic powder

Directions:

1.   Preheat a mini waffle iron and then grease it.

2.   In a medium bowl, place all ingredients and mix until well combined.

3.   Place 1/of the mixture into preheated waffle iron and cook for about 4-5 minutes or until golden brown.

4.   Repeat with the remaining mixture.

5.   Serve warm.

Nutrition value per Servings:

Calories: 95 Fat: 5.8g Carbohydrates: 2.2g Sugar: 0.3g Protein: 8g

Turkey Chaffles

Servings: 4

Cooking Time: 16 Minutes

Ingredients:

½ cup cooked turkey meat, chopped 2 organic eggs, beaten

½ cup Parmesan cheese, grated

½ cup Mozzarella, shredded

¼ teaspoon poultry seasoning

¼ teaspoon onion powder

Directions:

1.   Preheat a mini waffle iron and then grease it.

2.   In a medium bowl, place all ingredients and mix until well combined.

3.   Place ¼ of the mixture into preheated waffle iron and cook for about 4 minutes or until golden brown.

4.   Repeat with the remaining mixture.

5.   Serve warm.

Nutrition value per Servings:

Calories: 108 Fat: 1g Carbohydrates: 0.5g Sugar: 0.2g Protein: 12.9g

Pepperoni Chaffles

Servings: 1

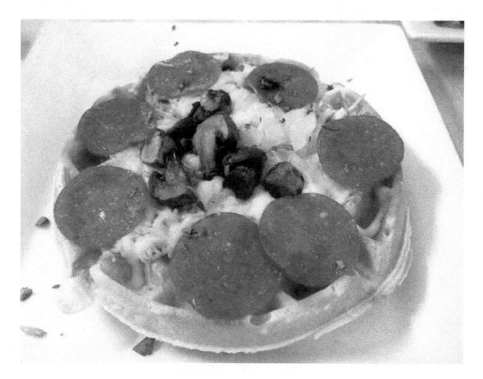

Cooking Time: 5 Minutes

Ingredients:

1   organic egg, beaten

½ cup Mozzarella cheese, shredded

2   tablespoons turkey pepperoni slice, chopped

1 tablespoon sugar-free pizza sauce ¼ teaspoon Italian seasoning

Directions:

1.   Preheat a waffle iron and then grease it.

2.   In a bowl, place all the ingredients and mix well.

3.   Place the mixture into preheated waffle iron and cook for about 5 minutes or until golden brown.

4.   Serve warm.

Nutrition value per Servings:

Calories: 119 Fat: 7.g Carbohydrates: 2.7g Sugar: 0.9g Protein: 10.3g

Hot Sauce Jalapeño Chaffles

Servings: 2

Cooking Time: 8 Minutes

Ingredients:

½ cup plus 2 teaspoons Cheddar cheese, shredded and divided 1 organic egg, beaten

6 jalapeño pepper slices

¼ teaspoon hot sauce Pinch of salt Directions:

1.   Preheat a mini waffle iron and then grease it.

2.   In a bowl, place ½ cup of cheese and remaining ingredients and mix until well combined.

3.   Place about 1 teaspoon of cheese in the bottom of the waffle maker for about seconds before adding the mixture.

4.   Place half of the mixture into preheated waffle iron and cook for about 3- minutes or until golden brown.

5.   Repeat with the remaining cheese and mixture.

6.   Serve warm.

Nutrition value per Servings:

Calories: 153 Fat: 12.2g Carbohydrates: 0.7g Sugar: 0.4g
Protein: 10.3g

Garlic Herb Blend Seasoning Chaffles

Servings: 2

Cooking Time: 8 Minutes

Ingredients:

1 large organic egg, beaten

¼ cup Parmesan cheese, shredded

¼ cup Mozzarella cheese, shredded

½ tablespoon butter, melted

1 teaspoon garlic herb blend seasoning Salt, to taste

Directions:

1.   Preheat a mini waffle iron and then grease it.

2.   In a bowl, place all the ingredients and beat until well combined.

3.   Place half of the mixture into preheated waffle iron and cook for about 4 minutes or until golden brown.

4.   Repeat with the remaining mixture.

5.   Serve warm.

Nutrition value per Servings:

Calories: 115 Fat: 8.8g Carbohydrates: 1.2g Sugar: 0.2g Protein: 8g

Protein Cheddar Chaffles

Servings: 8

Cooking Time: 48 Minutes

Ingredients:

½ cup golden flax seeds meal ½ cup almond flour 2 tablespoons unflavored whey protein powder

1   teaspoon organic baking powder Salt and ground black pepper, to taste

¾ cup cheddar cheese, shredded 1/3 cup unsweetened almond milk

2   tablespoons unsalted butter, melted 2 large organic eggs, beaten Directions:

1.   Preheat a mini waffle iron and then grease it.

2.   In a large bowl, add flax seeds meal, flour, protein powder, baking powder, and mix well.

3.   Stir in the cheddar cheese.

4.   In another bowl, add the remaining ingredients and beat until well combined.

5.   Add the egg mixture into the bowl with flax seeds meal mixture and mix until well combined.

6.   Place desired amount of the mixture into preheated waffle iron.

7.   Cook for about 4-6 minutes.

8.   Repeat with the remaining mixture.

9.   Serve warm. Nutrition value:

Calories 187 Fat 14.5 g Carbs 4.9 g Sugar 0.4 g Protein 8 g

Cheese-Free Breakfast Chaffle

Servings: 1

Cooking Time: 12 Minutes

Ingredients:

1   egg

½ cup almond milk ricotta, finely shredded. 1 tbsp almond flour

2   tbsp butter

Directions:

1.   Mix the egg, almond flour and ricotta in a small bowl.

2.   Separate the chaffle batter into two and cook each for 4 minutes.

3.   Melt the butter and pour on top of the chaffles.

4.   Put them back in the pan and cook on each side for 2 minutes.

5.   Remove from the pan and allow them sit for 2 minutes.

6.   Enjoy while still crispy Nutrition value:

Calories 530 ; Fats: 50 g ; Carbs: 3 g ; Protein: 23 g

Savory Bagel Seasoning Chaffles

Servings:4

Cooking Time: 5 Minutes

Ingredients:

2 tbsps. everything bagel seasoning 2 eggs

1 cup mozzarella cheese 1/2 cup grated parmesan Directions:

1.   Preheat the square waffle maker and grease with cooking spray.

2.   Mix eggs, mozzarella cheese and grated cheese in a bowl.

3.   Pour half of the batter in the waffle maker.

4.   Sprinkle 1 tbsp. of the everything bagel seasoning over batter.

5.   Close the lid.

6.   Cook chaffles for about 3-4 minutes.

7.   Repeat with the remaining batter.

8.   Serve hot and enjoy! Nutrition value per Servings:

Calories 170 Fat: 13 g ; Carbs: 2 g ; Protein: 11 g

Dried Herbs Chaffles

Servings: 2

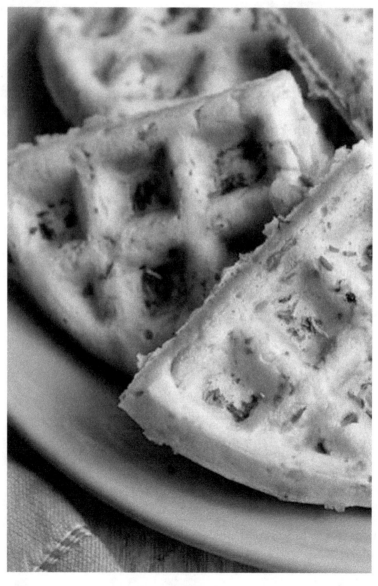

Cooking Time: 8 Minutes

Ingredients:

1 organic egg, beaten

½ cup Cheddar cheese, shredded 1 tablespoon almond flour

Pinch of dried thyme, crushed

Pinch of dried rosemary, crushed

Directions:

1.   Preheat a mini waffle iron and then grease it.

2.   In a bowl, place all the ingredients and beat until well combined.

3.   Place half of the mixture into preheated waffle iron and cook for about 4 minutes or until golden brown.

4.   Repeat with the remaining mixture.

5.   Serve warm.

Nutrition value per Servings:

Calories: 112 Fat: 13.4g Carbohydrates: 1.3g Sugar: 0.4g Protein: 9.8g

Cookie Dough Chaffle

Servings:4

Cooking Time:7-9 Minutes

Ingredients:

Batter 4 eggs

¼ cup heavy cream

1 teaspoon vanilla extract ¼ cup stevia 6 tablespoons coconut flour

1   teaspoon baking powder Pinch of salt

¼ cup unsweetened chocolate chips

Other

2   tablespoons cooking spray to brush the waffle maker ¼ cup heavy cream, whipped

Directions:

1.   Preheat the waffle maker.

2.   Add the eggs and heavy cream to a bowl and stir in the vanilla extract, stevia, coconut flour, baking powder, and salt. Mix until just combined.

3.   Stir in the chocolate chips and combine.

4.   Brush the heated waffle maker with cooking spray and add a few tablespoons of the batter.

5.   Close the lid and cook for about 7-8 minutes depending on your waffle maker.

6.   Serve with whipped cream on top. Nutrition value per Servings:

Calories 30 fat 32.3 g carbs 12.6 g, sugar 0.5 g, Protein 9 g

Thanksgiving Pumpkin Spice Chaffle

Servings:4

Cooking Time:5minutes

Ingredients:

1   cup egg whites

¼ cup pumpkin puree

2   tsps. pumpkin pie spice

2 tsps. coconut flour ½ tsp. vanilla 1 tsp. baking powder

1 tsp. baking soda

1/8 tsp cinnamon powder

1 cup mozzarella cheese, grated 1/2 tsp. garlic powder

Directions:

1.   Switch on your square waffle maker. Spray with non-stick spray.

2.   Beat egg whites with beater, until fluffy and white.

3.   Add pumpkin puree, pumpkin pie spice, coconut flour in egg whites and beat again.

4.   Stir in the cheese, cinnamon powder, garlic powder, baking soda, and powder.

5. Pour ½ of the batter in the waffle maker.

6. Close the maker and cook for about 3 minutes.

7. Repeat with the remaining batter.

8. Remove chaffles from the maker.

9. Serve hot and enjoy!

Nutrition value per Servings: Protein: 51% 66 kcal Fat: 41% 53 kcal

Carbohydrates: 8% kcal

Pumpkin Spice Chaffles

Servings: 2

Cooking Time: 14 Minutes

Ingredients:

1 egg, beaten

½ tsp pumpkin pie spice

½ cup finely grated mozzarella cheese 1 tbsp sugar-free pumpkin puree Directions:

1.   Preheat the waffle iron.

2.   In a medium bowl, mix all the ingredients.

3.   Open the iron, pour in half of the batter, close, and cook until crispy, 6 to 7 minutes.

4.   Remove the chaffle onto a plate and set aside.

5.   Make another chaffle with the remaining batter.

6.   Allow cooling and serve afterward. Nutrition value:

Calories 90 Fats 6.46g Carbs 1.98g Protein 5.94g

Chaffle Fruit Snacks

Servings: 2

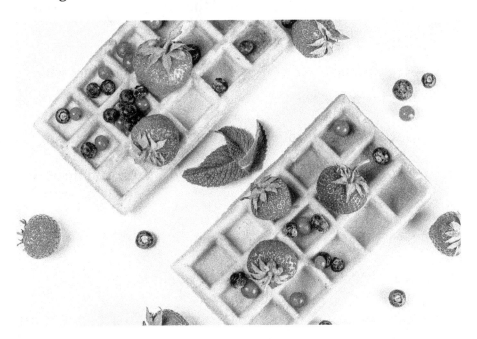

Cooking Time: 14 Minutes

Ingredients:

1 egg, beaten

½ cup finely grated cheddar cheese

½ cup Greek yogurt for topping

8 raspberries and blackberries for topping

Directions:

1.   Preheat the waffle iron.

2.   Mix the egg and cheddar cheese in a medium bowl.

3.   Open the iron and add half of the mixture. Close and cook until crispy, 7 minutes.

4.   Remove the chaffle onto a plate and make another with the remaining mixture.

5.   Cut each chaffle into wedges and arrange on a plate.

6.   Top each waffle with a tablespoon of yogurt and then two berries.

7.   Serve afterward. Nutrition value:

Calories 207 Fats 15.29g Carbs 4.36g Protein 12.91g

Open-Faced Ham & Green Bell Pepper Chaffle Sandwich

Servings: 2

Cooking Time: 10 Minutes

Ingredients:

2 slices ham Cooking spray

1 green bell pepper, sliced into strips 2 slices cheese

1 tablespoon black olives, pitted and sliced 2 basic chaffles

Directions:

1.	Cook the ham in a pan coated with oil over medium heat.

2.	Next, cook the bell pepper.

3.	Assemble the open-faced sandwich by topping each chaffle with ham and cheese, bell pepper and olives.

4.	Toast in the oven until the cheese has melted a little. Nutrition value:

Calories 36 Fat 24.6g Carbohydrate 8g Protein 24.5g Sugars 6.3g

Christmas Morning Choco Chaffle Cake

Servings:8

Cooking Time:5minutes

Ingredients:

8 keto chocolate square chaffles 2 cups peanut butter

16 oz. raspberries

Directions:

1.	Assemble chaffles in layers.

2.	Spread peanut butter in each layer.

3.	Top with raspberries.

4.	Enjoy cake on Christmas morning with keto coffee!
Nutrition value per Servings:

Calories 170 Fat: 13 g ; Carbs: 2 g ; Protein: 11 g

Lt Chaffle Sandwich

Servings: 2

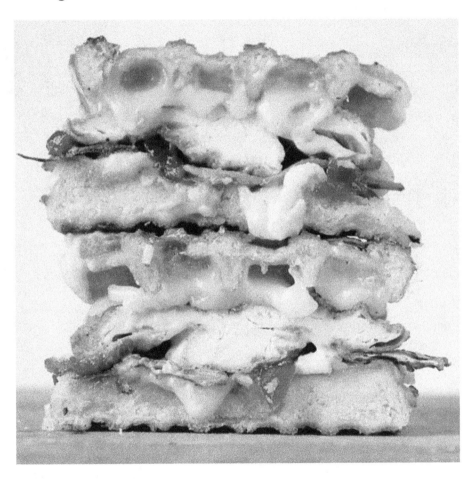

Cooking Time: 15 Minutes

Ingredients:

Cooking spray 4 slices bacon

1 tablespoon mayonnaise

4 basic chaffles

2 lettuce leaves

2 tomato slices

Directions:

1.   Coat your pan with foil and place it over medium heat.

2.   Cook the bacon until golden and crispy.

3.   Spread mayo on top of the chaffle.

4.   Top with the lettuce, bacon and tomato.

5.   Top with another chaffle. Nutrition value:

Calories 238 Fat 18.4g Carbohydrate 3g Protein 14.3g Sugars 0.9g

Mozzarella Peanut Butter Chaffle

Servings: 2

Cooking Time: 15 Minutes

Ingredients:

1 egg, lightly beaten 2 tbsp peanut butter 2 tbsp Swerve

1/2 cup mozzarella cheese, shredded

Directions:

1.   Preheat your waffle maker.

2.   In a bowl, mix egg, cheese, Swerve, and peanut butter until well combined.

3.   Spray waffle maker with cooking spray.

4.   Pour half batter in the hot waffle maker and cook for minutes or until golden brown. Repeat with the remaining batter.

5.   Serve and enjoy. Nutrition value:

Calories 150 Fat 11.5 g Carbohydrates 5.g Sugar 1.7 g Protein 8.8 g

Double Decker Chaffle

Servings:2

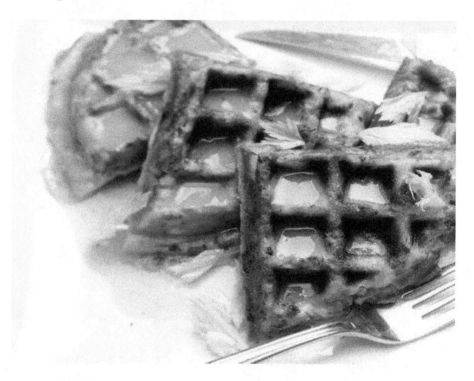

Cooking Time: 10 Minutes

Ingredients:

1 large egg

1 cup shredded cheese TOPPING

1   keto chocolate ball 2 oz. cranberries

2   oz. blueberries

4 oz. cranberries puree

Directions:

1.   Make 2 minutesi dash waffles.

2.   Put cranberries and blueberries in the freezer for about hours.

3.   For serving, arrange keto chocolate ball between 2 chaffles.

4.   Top with frozen berries,

5.   Serve and enjoy! Nutrition value per Servings:

Calories 170 Fat: 13 g ; Carbs: 2 g ; Protein: 11 g

Cinnamon And Vanilla Chaffle

Servings:4

Cooking Time:7-9 Minutes

Ingredients:

Batter 4 eggs

4 ounces sour cream

1 teaspoon vanilla extract

1 teaspoon cinnamon ¼ cup stevia 5 tablespoons coconut flour

Other

2 tablespoons coconut oil to brush the waffle maker

½ teaspoon cinnamon for garnishing the chaffles

Directions:

1. Preheat the waffle maker.

2. Add the eggs and sour cream to a bowl and stir with a wire whisk until just combined.

3. Add the vanilla extract, cinnamon, and stevia and mix until combined.

4. Stir in the coconut flour and stir until combined.

5.   Brush the heated waffle maker with coconut oil and add a few tablespoons of the batter.

6.   Close the lid and cook for about 7-8 minutes depending on your waffle maker.

7.   Serve and enjoy. Nutrition value per Servings:

Calories 224, fat 11 g, carbs 8.4 g, sugar 0.5 g, Protein 7.7 g

New Year Cinnamon Chaffle With Coconut Cream

Servings:2

Cooking Time:5minutes

Ingredients:

2 large eggs

1/8 cup almond flour

1 tsp. cinnamon powder 1 tsp. sea salt

1/2 tsp. baking soda

1 cup shredded mozzarella FOR TOPPING 2 tbsps. coconut cream

1   tbsp. unsweetened chocolate sauce

Directions:

1.   Preheat waffle maker according to the manufacturer's directions.

2.   Mix recipe ingredients in a mixing bowl.

3.   Add cheese and mix well.

4.   Pour about ½ cup mixture into the waffle maker's center and cook for about 2-3 minutes until golden and crispy.

5.   Repeat with the remaining batter.

6.   For serving, coat coconut cream over chaffles. Drizzle chocolate sauce over chaffle.

7.   Freeze chaffle in the freezer for about10 minutes.

8.   Serve on Christmas morning and enjoy! Nutrition value per Servings:

Calories 170 Fat: 13 g ; Carbs: 2 g ; Protein: 11 g

Chaffles And Ice-Cream Platter

Servings: 2

Cooking Time:5 minutes

Ingredients:

2   keto brownie chaffles

2 scoop vanilla keto ice cream 8 oz. strawberries, sliced

keto chocolate sauce

Directions:

1.   Arrange chaffles, ice-cream, strawberries slice in serving plate.

2.   Drizzle chocolate sauce on top.

3.   Serve and enjoy! Nutrition value per Servings:

Calories 170 Fat: 13 g ; Carbs: 2 g ; Protein: 11 g

Choco Chip Pumpkin Chaffle

Servings: 2

Cooking Time: 15 Minutes

Ingredients:

1 egg, lightly beaten 1 tbsp almond flour

1 tbsp unsweetened chocolate chips 1/4 tsp pumpkin pie spice 2 tbsp Swerve

1   tbsp pumpkin puree

1/2 cup mozzarella cheese, shredded

Directions:

1.   Preheat your waffle maker.

2.   In a small bowl, mix egg and pumpkin puree.

3.   Add pumpkin pie spice, Swerve, almond flour, and cheese and mix well.

4.   Stir in chocolate chips.

5.   Spray waffle maker with cooking spray.

6.   Pour half batter in the hot waffle maker and cook for 4 minutes. Repeat with the remaining batter.

7.   Serve and enjoy. Nutrition value:

Calories 130 Fat 9.2 g Carbohydrates 5.9 g Sugar 0.6 g Protein 6.6 g

Sausage & Pepperoni Chaffle Sandwich

Servings: 4

Cooking Time: 10 Minutes

Ingredients:

Cooking spray

2   cervelat sausage, sliced into rounds 12 pieces pepperoni

6 mushroom slices

4 teaspoons mayonnaise 4 big white onion rings 4 basic chaffles
Directions:

1.   Spray your skillet with oil.

2.   Place over medium heat.

3.   Cook the sausage until brown on both sides.

4.   Transfer on a plate.

5.   Cook the pepperoni and mushrooms for 2 minutes.

6.   Spread mayo on top of the chaffle.

7.   Top with the sausage, pepperoni, mushrooms and onion
rings.

8.   Top with another chaffle. Nutrition value:

Calories 373 Fat 24.4g Carbohydrate 28g Protein 8.1g Sugars 4.5g

Maple Chaffle

Servings: 2

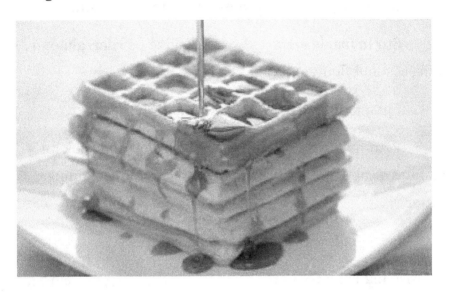

Cooking Time: 15 Minutes

Ingredients:

1   egg, lightly beaten

2   2 egg whites

1/2 tsp maple extract

2   tsp Swerve

1/2 tsp baking powder, gluten-free

2 tbsp almond milk

2 tbsp coconut flour

Directions:

1.   Preheat your waffle maker.

2.   In a bowl, whip egg whites until stiff peaks form.

3.   Stir in maple extract, Swerve, baking powder, almond milk, coconut flour, and egg.

4.   Spray waffle maker with cooking spray.

5.   Pour half batter in the hot waffle maker and cook for 3-minutes or until golden brown. Repeat with the remaining batter.

6.   Serve and enjoy. Nutrition value:

Calories 122 Fat 6.6 g Carbohydrates 9 g Sugar 1 g Protein 7 g

Fruity Vegan Chaffles

Servings:2

Cooking Time:5minutes

Ingredients:

1 tbsp. chia seeds

2 tbsps. warm water

¼ cup low carb vegan cheese

2 tbsps. strawberry puree

2 tbsps. Greek yogurt

pinch of salt

Directions:

1. Preheat minutesi waffle maker to medium-high heat.

2. In a small bowl, mix chia seeds and water and let it stand for few minutes to be thickened.

3. Mix the rest of the ingredients in chia seed egg and mix well.

4. Spray waffle machine with cooking spray.

5. Pour vegan waffle batter into the center of the waffle iron.

6. Close the waffle maker and cook chaffles for about 3-5 minutes.

7. Once cooked, remove from the maker and serve with berries on top. Nutrition value per Servings:

Calories: 145 Fat: 9.4g Carbohydrates: 1g Sugar: 0.2g Protein: 14.3g

Almonds And Flaxseeds Chaffles

Servings:2

Cooking Time:5minutes

Ingredients:

1/4 cup coconut flour

1 tsp. stevia

1 tbsp. ground flaxseed

2 1/4 tsp baking powder 1/2 cup almond milk

3 1/4 tsp vanilla extract

1/ cup low carb vegan cheese

Directions:

1. Mix flaxseed in warm water and set aside.

2. Add in the remaining ingredients.

3. Switch on waffle iron and grease with cooking spray.Pour the batter in the waffle machine and close the lid.

4. Cook the chaffles for about 3-4 minutes.

5. Once cooked, remove from the waffle machine.

6. Serve with berries and enjoy! Nutrition value per Servings: Calories 42 fat 32.8 g, carbs 9.5 g, sugar 1.1 g, Protein 25.7 g

Vegan Chocolate Chaffles

Servings:2

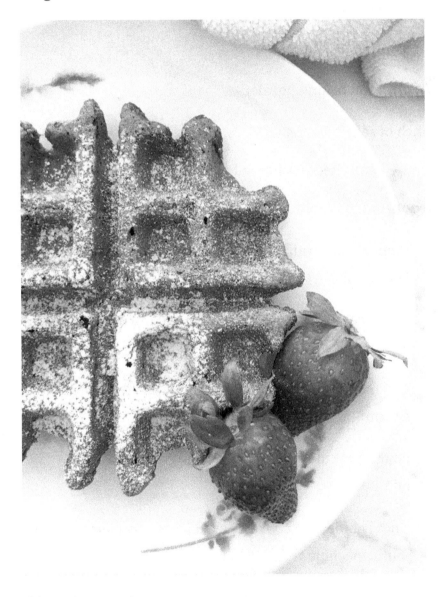

Cooking Time: 5minutes

Ingredients:

1/2 cupcoconut flour

3 tbsps. cocoa powder

4 tbsps. whole psyllium husk

5 1/2 teaspoon baking powder

6 pinch of salt

1/2 cup vegan cheese, softened 1/4 cup coconut milk

Directions:

1. Prepare your waffle iron according to the manufacturer's Directions.

2. Mix coconut flour, cocoa powder, baking powder, salt and husk in a bowl and set aside.

3. Add melted cheese and milk and mix well. Let it stand for a few minutes before cooking.

4. Pour batter in waffle machine and cook for about 3-minutes.

5. Once chaffles are cooked, carefully remove them from the waffle machine.

6. Serve with vegan icecream and enjoy!

Nutrition value per Servings:

Calories 196, fat 16 g, carbs 4 g, sugar 1 g, Protein 10.8 g

Vegan Chaffles With Flaxseed

Servings:2

Cooking Time: 5minutes

Ingredients:

1 tbsp. flaxseed meal

2 2 tbsps. warm water

¼ cup low carb vegan cheese

¼ cup chopped minutest pinch of salt

3 oz. blueberries chunks

Directions:

1. Preheat waffle maker to medium-high heat and grease with cooking spray.

2. Mix flaxseed meal and warm water and set aside to be thickened.

3. After 5 minutes' mix together all ingredients in flax egg.

4. Pour vegan waffle batter into the center of the waffle iron.

5. Close the waffle maker and let cook for 3-minutes

6. Once cooked, remove the vegan chaffle from the waffle maker and serve. Nutrition value per Servings:

Calories 42 fat 32.8 g, carbs 9.5 g, sugar 1.1 g, Protein 25.7 g

Asparagus Chaffle

Servings:4

Cooking Time:15 Minutes

Ingredients:

Batter 4 eggs

1½ cups grated mozzarella cheese

½ cup grated parmesan cheese

1 cup boiled asparagus, chopped

2 Salt and pepper to taste

¼ cup almond flour

3 teaspoons baking powder

4 tablespoons cooking spray to brush the waffle maker

5 ¼ cup Greek yogurt for serving

¼ cup chopped almonds for serving

Directions:

1. Preheat the waffle maker.

2. Add the eggs, grated mozzarella, grated parmesan, asparagus, salt and pepper, almond flour and baking powder to a bowl.

3. Mix with a fork.

4. Brush the heated waffle maker with cooking spray and add a few tablespoons of the batter.

5. Close the lid and cook for about 7 minutes depending on your waffle maker.

6. Serve each chaffle with Greek yogurt and chopped almonds. Nutrition value per Servings:

Calories 316, fat 24.9 g, carbs 3 g, sugar 1.2 g, Protein 18.2 g

Rosemary Pork Chops On Chaffle

Servings:4 Cooking Time:15 Minutes

Ingredients:

4 eggs

3 cups grated mozzarella cheese

4 Salt and pepper to taste Pinch of nutmeg

2 tablespoons sour cream

5 tablespoons almond flour

6 2 teaspoons baking powder

7 Pork chops

2 tablespoons olive oil

1 pound pork chops

Salt and pepper to taste

1 teaspoon freshly chopped rosemary

2 tablespoons cooking spray to brush the waffle maker 2 tablespoons freshly chopped basil for decoration

Directions:

1.   Preheat the waffle maker.

2. Add the eggs, mozzarella cheese, salt and pepper, nutmeg, sour cream, almond flour and baking powder to a bowl.

3. Mix until combined.

4. Brush the heated waffle maker with cooking spray and add a few tablespoons of the batter.

5. Close the lid and cook for about 7 minutes depending on your waffle maker.

6. Meanwhile, heat the butter in a nonstick grill pan and season the pork chops with salt and pepper and freshly chopped rosemary.

7. Cook the pork chops for about 4-5 minutes on each side.

8. Serve each chaffle with a pork chop and sprinkle some freshly chopped basil on top.

Nutrition value per Servings:

Calories 666, fat 55.2 g, carbs 4.8 g, sugar 0.4 g, Protein 37.5 g

Classic Beef Chaffle

Servings:4

Cooking Time:10 Minutes

Ingredients:

Batter

½ pound ground beef

4 eggs

4 ounces cream cheese

1 cup grated mozzarella cheese

2 Salt and pepper to taste

3 1 clove garlic, minced

½ teaspoon freshly chopped rosemary

4 tablespoons butter to brush the waffle maker

5 ¼ cup sour cream

6 2 tablespoons freshly chopped parsley for garnish

Directions:

1. Preheat the waffle maker.

2. Add the ground beef, eggs, cream cheese, grated mozzarella cheese, salt and pepper, minced garlic and freshly chopped rosemary to a bowl.

3. Brush the heated waffle maker with butter and add a few tablespoons of the batter.

4. Close the lid and cook for about 8-10 minutes depending on your waffle maker.

5. Serve each chaffle with a tablespoon of sour cream and freshly chopped parsley on top.

6. Serve and enjoy.

Nutrition value per Servings:

Calories 368, fat 24 g, carbs 2.1 g, sugar 0.4 g, Protein 27.4 g

Sloppy Joe Chaffle

Servings: 2

Cooking Time: 20 Minutes

Ingredients:

Chaffle:

1 large egg (beaten)

1/8 tsp onion powder

1 tbsp almond flour

½ cup shredded mozzarella cheese

1 tsp nutmeg

¼ tsp baking powder Sloppy Joe Filling:

2 tsp olive oil

1 pounds ground beef

1 celery stalk (chopped)

2 2 tbsp ketch up

3 tsp Worcestershire sauce 1 small onions (chopped)

1 green bell pepper (chopped)

1 tbsp sugar free maple syrup

1 cup tomato sauce (7.9 ounce)

2 garlic cloves (minced)

½ tsp salt or to taste

½ tsp ground black pepper or to taste

Directions:

1.   For the chaffle:

2.   Plug the waffle maker and preheat it. Spray it with non-stick spray.

3.   Combine the baking powder, nutmeg, flour and onion powder in a mixing bowl. Add the eggs and mix.

4.   Add the cheese and mix until the ingredients are well combined and you have formed a smooth batter.

5.   Pour the batter into the waffle maker and spread it out to the edges of the waffle maker to cover all the holes on it.

6.   Close the waffle lid and cook for about 5 minutes or according to waffle maker's settings.

7.   After the cooking cycle, remove the chaffle from the waffle maker with a plastic or silicone utensil. Transfer the chaffle to a wire rack to cool.

8.   For the sloppy joe filling:

9. Heat a large skillet over medium to high heat.

10. Add the ground beef and saute until the beef is browned.

11. Use a slotted spoon to transfer the ground beef to a paper towel lined plate to drain. Drain all the grease in the skillet.

12. Add the olive oil to the skillet and heat it.

13. Add the onions, green pepper, celery and garlic. Saute until the veggies are tender, stirring often to prevent burning.

14. Stir in the tomato sauce, Worcestershire sauce, ketchup, maple syrup, salt and pepper.

15. Add the browned beef and bring the mixture to a boil. Reduce the heat and simmer for about 10 minutes.

16. Remove the skillet from heat.

17. Scoop the sloppy joe into the chaffles and enjoy. Nutrition value per Servings:

Calories 168 Fat 15.5g Carbohydrate 1.6g Protein 5.4g Sugars 0.6g

Choco Peanut Butter Chaffle

Servings: 2

Cooking Time: 10 Minutes

Ingredients:

<u>Filling:</u>

4 tbsp all-natural peanut butter

5 2 tsp swerve sweetener

1 tsp vanilla extract

2 tbsp heavy cream <u>Chaffle:</u>

¼ tsp baking powder

1 tbsp unsweetened cocoa powder

4 tsp almond flour

½ tsp vanilla extract

1 tbsp granulated swerve sweetener

1 large egg (beaten)

1 tbsp heavy cream

Directions:

1. For the chaffle:

2.   Plug the waffle maker and preheat it. Spray it with a non-stick spray.

3.   In a large mixing bowl, combine the almond flour, cocoa powder, baking powder and swerve.

4.   Add the egg, vanilla extract and heavy cream. Mix until the ingredients are well combined and you form a smooth batter.

5.   Pour some of the batter into the preheated waffle maker. Spread out the batter to the waffle maker's edges to cover all the holes on the waffle iron.

6.   Close the lid of the waffle iron and bake for about 5 minutes or according to waffle maker's settings.

7.   After the baking cycle, use a plastic or silicone utensil to remove the chaffle from the waffle maker.

8.   Repeat step 4 to 6 until you have cooked all the batter into chaffles.

9.   Transfer the chaffles to a wire rack and let the chaffles cool completely.

10.   For the filling:

11. Combine the vanilla, swerve, heavy cream and peanut butter in a bowl. Mix until the ingredients are well combined.

12. Spread the peanut butter frosting over the chaffles and serve.

13. Enjoy.

Nutrition value per Servings:

Calories 158 Fat 18.5g Carbohydrate 2.6g Protein 7.4g Sugars 0.6g

Zucchini Bacon Chaffles

Servings: 2

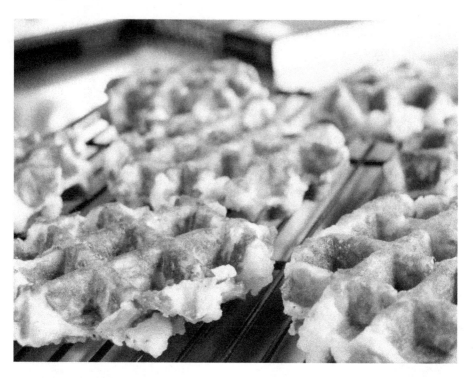

Cooking Time: 12 Minutes

Ingredients:

1 cup grated zucchini

1 tbsp bacon bits (finely chopped)

¼ cup shredded mozzarella cheese

½ cup shredded parmesan

½ tsp salt or to taste

½ tsp ground black pepper or to taste

½ tsp onion powder

¼ tsp nutmeg

2 eggs

Directions:

1.   Add ¼ tsp salt to the grated zucchini and let it sit for about 5 minutes.

2.   Put the grated zucchini in a clean towel and squeeze out excess water.

3.   Plug the waffle maker and preheat it. Spray it with non-stick spray.

4.   Break the eggs into a mixing bowl and beat.

5.   Add the grated zucchini, bacon bit, nutmeg, onion powder, pepper, salt and mozzarella.

6.   Add ¾ of the parmesan cheese. You have to set aside some parmesan cheese.

7.   Mix until the ingredients are well combined.

8.   Fill the preheated waffle maker with the batter and spread out the batter to the edge to cover all the holes on the waffle maker.

9.   Close the waffle maker lid and cook until the chaffle is golden brown and crispy. The zucchini chaffle may take longer than other chaffles to get crispy.

10.   After the baking cycle, use a plastic or silicone utensil to remove the chaffle from the waffle maker.

11.   Repeat step 8 to 10 until you have cooked all the batter into chaffles.

12.   Serve and enjoy.

Spinach Artichoke Chaffle With Bacon

Servings: 2

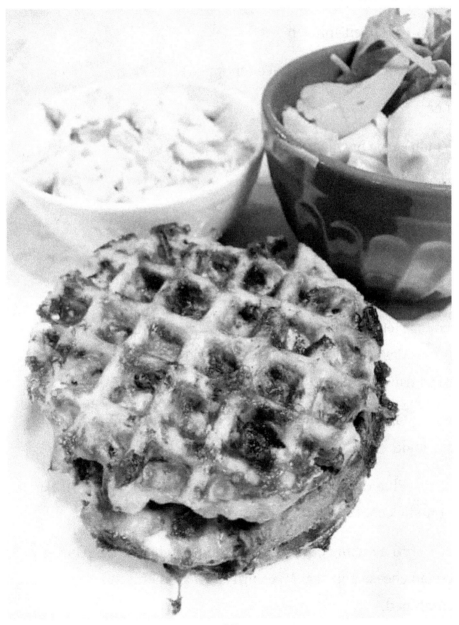

Cooking Time: 8 Minutes

Ingredients:

4 slices of bacon

½ cup chopped spinach

1/3 cup marinated artichoke (chopped)

1 egg

¼ tsp garlic powder

¼ tsp smoked paprika

3 tbsp cream cheese (softened)

4 1/3 cup shredded mozzarella

5 Directions:

1.   Heat a frying pan and add the bacon slices. Sear until both sides of the bacon slices are browned. Use a slotted spoon to transfer the bacon to a paper towel line plate to drain.

2.   Once the bacon slices are cool, chop them into bits and set aside.

3.   Plug the waffle maker to preheat it and spray it with a non-stick cooking spray.

4.   In a mixing bowl, combine mozzarella, garlic, paprika, cream cheese and egg. Mix until the ingredients are well combined.

5.   Add the spinach, artichoke and bacon bit. Mix until they are well incorporated.

6.   Pour an appropriate amount of the batter into the waffle maker and spread it to the edges to cover all the holes on the waffle maker.

7.   Close the waffle maker and cook 4 minutes or more, according to your waffle maker's settings.

8.   After the cooking cycle, use a silicone or plastic utensil to remove the chaffle from the waffle maker.

9.   Repeat step 6 to 8 until you have cooked all the batter into chaffles.

10.   Serve and top with sour cream as desired. Nutrition value per Servings:

Calories 258 Fat 16.5g Carbohydrate 1.7g Protein 8.2g Sugars 0.6g

Chocolate Cannoli Chaffle

Servings: 4

Cooking Time: 10 Minutes

Ingredients:

Cannoli Topping:

2 tbsp granulated swerve 4 tbsp cream cheese

¼ tsp vanilla extract

¼ tsp cinnamon

6 tbsp ricotta cheese 1 tsp lemon juice Chaffle:

3 tbsp almond flour 1 tbsp swerve

1 egg

1/8 tsp baking powder 3/4 tbsp butter (melted)

½ tsp nutmeg

1 tbsp sugar free chocolate chips 1/8 tsp vanilla extract

Directions:

1.   Plug the waffle maker to preheat it and spray it with a non-stick spray.

2.   In a mixing bowl, whisk together the egg, butter and vanilla extract.

3.   In another mixing bowl, combine the almond flour, baking powder, nutmeg, chocolate chips and swerve.

4.   Pour the egg mixtura into the flour mixture and mix until the ingredients are well combined and you have formed a smooth batter.

5.   Fill your waffle maker with an appropriate amount of the batter and spread out the batter to the edged to cover all the holes on the waffle maker.

6.   Close the waffle maker and cook for about 4 minutes or according to waffle maker's settings.

7.   After the baking cycle, remove the chaffle from the waffle maker with a plastic or silicone utensil.

8.   Repeat step 5 to 7 until you have cooked all the batter into waffles.

9.   For the topping, pour the cream cheese into a blender and add the ricotta, lemon juice, cinnamon, vanilla and swerve sweetener. Blend until smooth and fluffy.

10.   Spread the cream over the chaffles and enjoy. Nutrition value per Servings:

Calories 208 Fat 18.5g Carbohydrate 1.7g Protein 4.2g Sugars 0.9g

Broccoli And Cheese Chaffle

Servings: 1

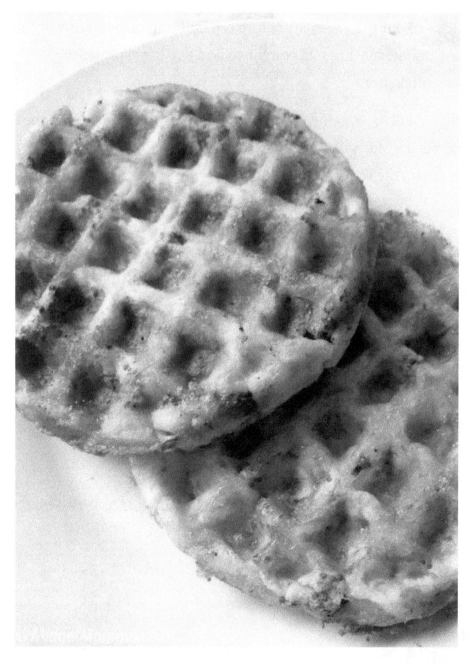

Cooking Time: 15 Minutes

Ingredients:

1/3 cup broccoli (finely chopped) ½ tsp oregano 1/8 tsp salt or to taste

1/8 tsp ground black pepper or to taste' ½ tsp garlic powder

½ tsp onion powder 1 egg (beaten)

4 tbsp shredded cheddar cheese

Directions:

1.   Plug the waffle maker to preheat it and spray it with a non-stick cooking spray.

2.   In a mixing bowl, combine the cheese, oregano, pepper, garlic, salt and onion. Add the egg and mix until the ingredients are well combined.

3.   Fold in the chopped broccoli.

4.   Pour an appropriate amount of the batter into your waffle maker and spread out the batter to the edges to cover all the holes on the waffle maker.

5.   Close the waffle maker and cook for about 6-8 until the chaffle is browned. Cook time may vary in some waffle makers.

6.   After the cooking cycle, use a silicone or plastic utensil to remove the chaffle from the waffle maker.

7.   Repeat step 4 to 6 until you have cooked all the batter into chaffles.

8.   Serve and top with sour cream as desired.

Nutrition value per Servings:

Calories 108 Fat 12.5g Carbohydrate 2.1g Protein 5.3g Sugars 1.1g

Carrot Cake Chaffle

Servings: 10

Cooking Time: 18 Minutes

Ingredients:

1 tbsp toasted pecans (chopped) 2 tbsp granulated swerve

1   tsp pumpkin spice 1 tsp baking powder

½ shredded carrots

2   tbsp butter (melted) 1 tsp cinnamon

1   tsp vanilla extract (optional)

2   tbsp heavy whipping cream ¾ cup almond flour 1 egg (beaten)

Butter cream cheese frosting:

½ cup cream cheese (softened)

¼ cup butter (softened)

½ tsp vanilla extract

¼ cup granulated swerve

Directions:

1.   Plug the chaffle maker to preheat it and spray it with a non-stick cooking spray.

2.   In a mixing bowl, combine the almond flour, cinnamon, carrot, pumpkin spice and swerve.

3.   In another mixing bowl, whisk together the eggs, butter, heavy whipping cream and vanilla extract.

4.   Pour the flour mixture into the egg mixture and mix until you form a smooth batter.

5.   Fold in the chopped pecans.

6.   Pour in an appropriate amount of the batter into your waffle maker and spread out the batter to the edges to cover all the holes on the waffle maker.

7.   Close the waffle maker and cook for about 3 minutes or according to your waffle maker's settings.

8.   After the cooking cycle, use a plastic or silicone utensil to remove the chaffle from the waffle maker.

9.   Repeat step 6 to 8 until you have cooked all the batter into chaffles.

10.   For the frosting, combine the cream cheese and cutter int a mixer and mix until well combined.

11.   Add the swerve and vanilla extract and slowly until the sweetener is well incorporated. Mix on high

until the frosting is fluffy.

12.   Place one chaffle on a flat surface and spread some cream frosting over it. Layer another chaffle over the first one a spread some cream over it too.

13.   Repeat step 12 until you have assembled all the chaffles into a cake.

14.   Cut and serve. Nutrition value per Servings:

Calories 208 Fat 13.5g Carbohydrate 0.7g Protein 8.2g Sugars 0.6g

Chaffles With Chocolate Balls

Servings:2

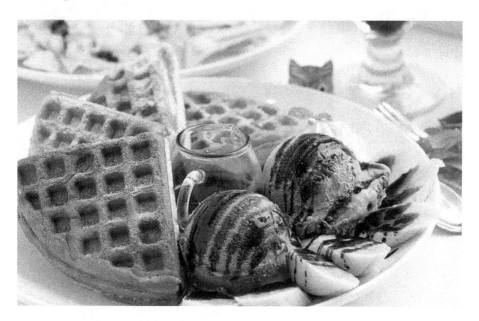

Cooking Time: 5 Minutes

Ingredients:

1/4 cup heavy cream

½ cup unsweetened cocoa powder

1/4 cup coconut meat

Chaffle ingredients:

1 egg

½ cup mozzarella cheese

Directions:

1.   Make 2 chaffles with chaffle ingredients.

2.   Meanwhile, mix all ingredients in a mixing bowl.

3.   Make two balls from the mixture and freeze in the freezer for about 2 hours until set.

4.   Serve with keto chaffles and enjoy! Nutrition value per Servings:

Calories 178 Fat 10.5g Carbohydrate 1.7g Protein 8.6g Sugars 1.6g

CPSIA information can be obtained
at www.ICGtesting.com
Printed in the USA
BVHW062016190321
602998BV00004B/76